BREAST CANCER REHABILITATION: USING SIMPLE LIFESTYLE STRATEGIES TO PREVENT THE OCCURRENCE AND REOCCURRENCE OF BREAST CANCER

By

Dr Loreb Robb

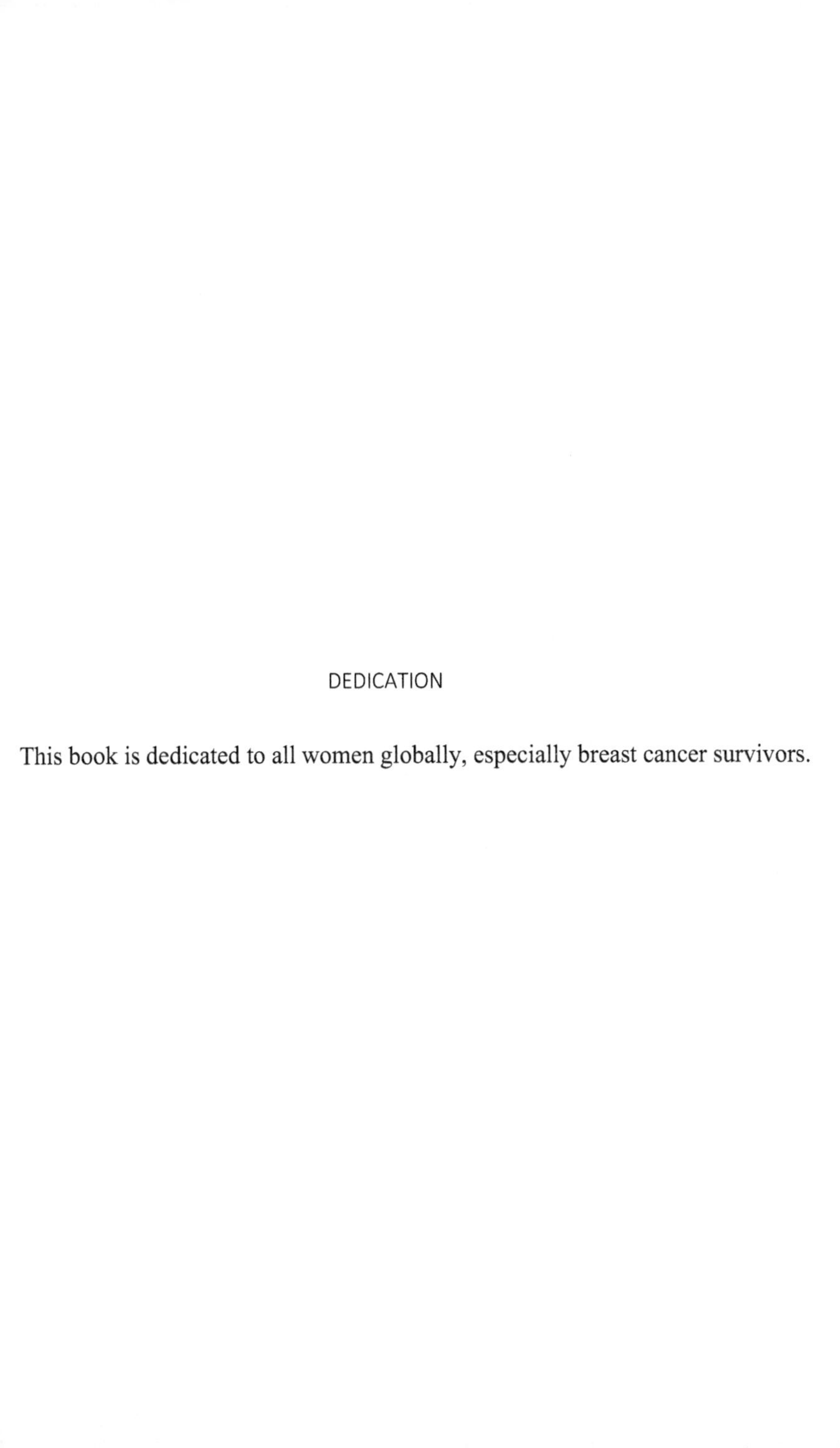

DEDICATION

This book is dedicated to all women globally, especially breast cancer survivors.

Contents

About the Author

Dr. Loreb Robb is a doctor in nursing practice with high knowledge and experience in midwifery practice and evidence-based studies in breast cancer rehabilitation with exercises. She has published many articles in health-related research studies. She presently authored this book entitled "BREAST CANCER REHABILITATION: USING SIMPLE LIFESTYLE TO PREVENT OCCURRENCE AND REOCCURRENCE OF BREAST CANCER" to help women navigate through this scary condition without being shattered and also live a high-quality life from diagnosis through treatment to survivorship. This article is an experience-riched book and will be beneficial to women globally as it will enable them to conquer breast cancer with its associated post-treatment complications in grand style.

Cancer of the breast is a subtype of a form of cancer that is distinguished by the presence of cells that are malignant in the breast tissue. Cancer of the breast is another term that can be used to describe a problem in which the cells of the breast increase in an uncontrolled manner. Typically, breast cancer is said to manifest in women aged 50 or above predominantly. It's critical to realize that it can influence young men, women, and other subgroups. When there is breast cancer, breast cells suffer an adverse shift, affecting the creation of cancer cells, and this is how breast cancer develops. As a result, these malignant cells escalate and grow into tumors. Breast cancer is seen as a complex disease with various symptoms and potential causes. It's important to note that having one or more of these symptoms does not necessarily mean a person has breast cancer, as other disease conditions can also cause these symptoms. To encourage early identification of breast cancer and to seek appropriate medical assistance, it is vital to be informed of both the symptoms and the causes of breast cancer, which can differ substantially. There is a significant difference in the incidence of breast cancer between men and women, but it is essential to be aware that breast cancer can affect both sexes. There are different types of cancer, each having its own peculiar symptoms and treatment protocol. It is also a necessity to decipher a normal breast tissue from an abnormal one to detect cancer of the breast as early as possible, as can be seen below.

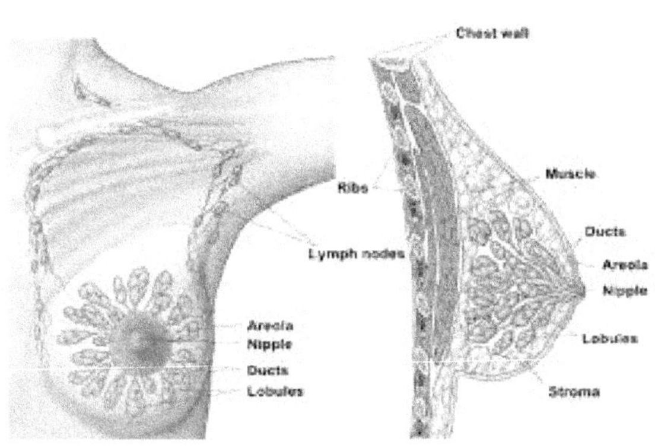

Figure 1:Normal breast tissues

Breast cancer

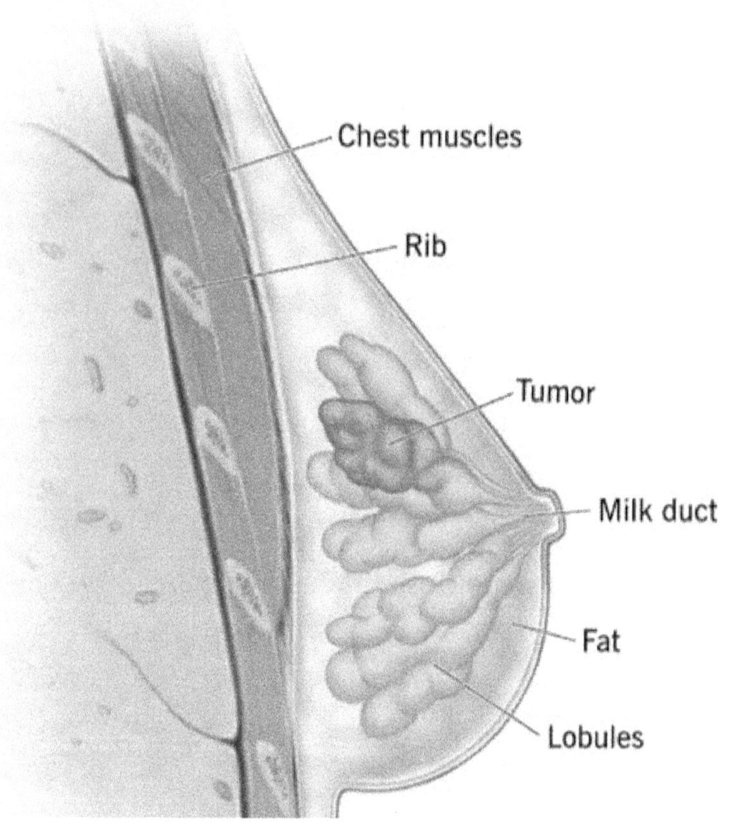

Figure 2: Breast with a tumor in-situ

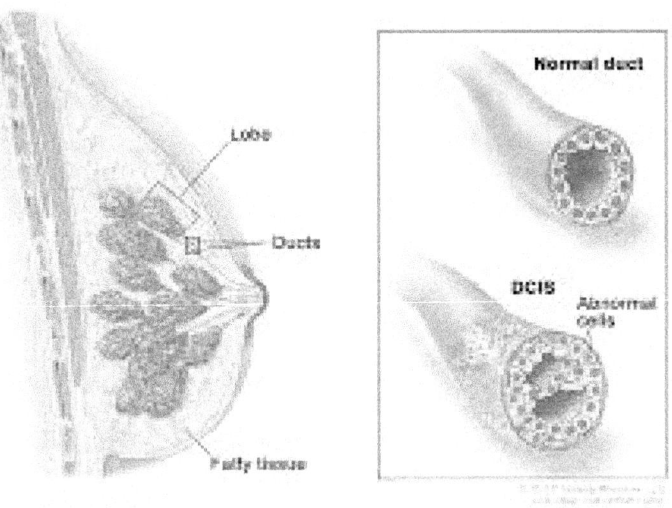

Figure 3: Ductal carcinoma in-situ

In addition to the preceding, the following are some of the symptoms of breast cancer:

1. Breast cancer is most commonly characterized by the presence of a lump or tumor in the breast or underarm region that does not cause any level of discomfort. A lump in the breast is another symptom that can be used to diagnose breast cancer. On the other hand, it is vital to remember that not all lumps are malignant and that breast lumps can also be caused by illnesses known to be benign.
2. Breast cancer can cause the breast to swell or shrink, as well as produce noteworthy changes in the breast's contour or shape. These changes can occur depending on the severity of the disease.
3. Alterations in the look of the Skin. Breast cancer can cause irregularities in the look of the skin, such as redness, dimpling, or puckering, which usually resembles an orange peel.
4. **Nipple Changes**: Changes in the nipple, such as inversion (turning inward), flaking, or discharge (other than breast milk), may indicate breast cancer.
5. **Nipple or Breast Pain**: Though uncommon, breast cancer can cause pain in the breast or nipple.
6. A thickened area in or near the chest or underarm may also suffice.
7. An area that isn't precisely equivalent to another location on either chest
8. Visible changes in the shape or position of the areola may suffix.
9. Changes in the skin of the chest or the areola might be dimpled, puckered, layered, or fueled.

Breast cancer is a life-threatening disease and has been seen as the most common cancer affecting women. Early detection of the disease remains a critical element of breast cancer control, as at this stage, women can undergo diagnosis and recover. However, if detected late, there is little scope for recovery, and only palliative care is provided to the patients and their families. The primary cause of breast can not be attributed to any exact cause; hence, the cause can be said to be unknown but may be predisposed by the following;

1. **Age and Gender**: The likelihood of developing breast cancer is higher as one gets older, and of all the risk factors, being female is the most significant. The incidence of breast cancer in men is similar to that of women, but it is much less common.
2. **Family History and Genetics**: A family history of breast cancer, especially in first-degree relatives (mother, sister, daughter), and specific gene mutations can increase the risk of developing breast cancer.
3. **Personal History of Breast Cancer**: It is more likely that a person will acquire cancer in the other breast or experience a recurrence of cancer if they had previously been diagnosed with breast cancer in one of their breasts.
4. **Hormonal Factors**: Factors such as early menstruation, late menopause, and late or no pregnancies can influence breast cancer risk. Long-term use of hormone replacement therapy (HRT) may also increase the risk.
5. **Lifestyle and Environmental Factors**: Factors like obesity, a sedentary lifestyle, alcohol consumption, and exposure to certain environmental toxins may contribute to an increased risk of breast cancer.
6. **Radiation Exposure**: Previous chest radiation for other medical conditions, especially during adolescence, can increase the risk of breast cancer later in life.

The two types of **invasive carcinoma developing at the highest rates are invasive lobular carcinoma** and invasive ductal carcinoma. It is estimated that around 70–80 percent of all occurrences of breast cancer are caused by invasive ductal carcinoma. For more information, breast cancer can be divided into two distinct groups, which are as follows:

1. **One type of breast cancer that does not spread to other parts of the body is called ductal carcinoma in situ (DCIS).** This type of breast cancer is distinguished by the presence of abnormal cells in the lining of a breast duct, but the disease has not spread beyond the confines of the ductal area.
2. **Invasive ductal carcinoma,** also known as IDC, is the most prevalent form of breast cancer. It is caused by the invasion of cancer cells into the breast's surrounding tissues outside the ducts.
3. **It is possible for invasive lobular carcinoma,** also known as ILC, to spread to other regions of the breast. ILC begins in the milk-producing glands, also known as lobules.
4. **Triple Negative Subtype:** This subtype of breast cancer does not have receptors for estrogen, progesterone, or HER2. Generally speaking, it is more aggressive.
5. **Breast** cancer that is HER2-positive is characterized by an overexpression of the HER2 protein and has a tendency to grow more rapidly than other types of breast cancer. There is the possibility of targeted therapy.
6. **There is a rare and dangerous kind of breast cancer known as inflammatory** breast cancer. This type of breast cancer manifests itself with redness, warmth, and swelling of the breast.

If you notice changes in your breasts, it is not time to get scared but search. It is essential to see a doctor immediately to discover the problem, as all changes may not result from cancer. Even if the changes are not due to cancer, it is better to be safe than sorry. Early detection and treatment of breast cancer are essential for improving the chances of survival. That is why women need to get regular mammograms and breast examinations. The essence is to search, not scare.

Prevention of breast cancer

Women can prevent breast cancer by using the following necessary tools;

1. Eating a healthy and balanced meal.

2. Maintaining good body weight.

3. Reduce alcohol intake and completely get rid of smoking.

4. Exercise regularly (at least for 150munites per week).

5. Get a mammogram once a year(mandatory for women above the age of 40)

6. Go for a clinical breast examination and also a monthly self-breast examination

7. Moreover, breastfeeding also reduces the risk of getting breast cancer to a great extent.

Being diagnosed with breast cancer can be a challenging and emotionally demanding experience, both in terms of the practical and emotional aspects of coping with the diagnosis. The diagnosis of breast cancer is not a death sentence and should not be treated as one. Diagnosis of breast cancer can make the individual take the following actions, which may not have been possible ordinarily without breast cancer. After the shock of diagnosis, there are practical issues to deal with — will there be surgery? How invasive, and when? And after surgery (or sometimes before), will there be adjuvant treatments such as chemotherapy or radiation? Some of the things that may help in dealing with the diagnosis of breast cancer may include the following;

1. Opting for healthier alternatives

   Many people find that receiving a diagnosis of cancer enables them to concentrate on their health in ways that they may not have given much thought to in the past of their health. Are you able to engage in activities that could improve your health? Attempt to improve your diet or increase the amount of physical activity you get. Reduce the amount of alcohol you consume or quit smoking. Keeping your stress level under control is one example of something that could be helpful. Right now is a beautiful time to give some thought to making adjustments that could have a beneficial impact on your life for the rest of your life. Making these adjustments will not only help you feel better, but they will also improve your health.

2. Take action on the things that trouble you the most. Focus on the items with the most cause for concern. Get assistance with the ones that are more difficult for you. Ensure that your level of tension is kept to an absolute minimum. It is time to choose and choose the things that cause you stress and to avoid taking everything in without question.

3. Improve your eating habits: Maintaining a healthy diet can be challenging for anybody, but it can become even more challenging during and after cancer treatment. Your taste buds might be altered as a result of treatment. An issue that may arise is nausea. You might not desire to eat and lose weight even though you don't want to. On the other hand, you might have put on weight you cannot get rid of. All of these things have the potential to be incredibly annoying. If the treatment produces changes in your weight and difficulties with eating or taste, you should do all in your power to fix these issues and keep in mind that they typically improve over time. Meanwhile, consuming little quantities every two to three hours might be helpful until you feel better. It is also a good idea to inquire with your cancer team about the possibility of consulting a nutritionist who is a nutrition specialist and can provide suggestions on how to deal with the adverse effects of treatment. Establishing and maintaining healthy eating habits regularly is one of the most beneficial things you can do after cancer treatment. You'll be surprised by the long-term benefits of making relatively minor adjustments, such as increasing the range of nutritious meals you consume. In addition to having a multitude of other positive effects on one's health, achieving and maintaining a healthy weight, adhering to a healthy

diet, and reducing the amount of alcohol consumed can potentially reduce the risk of developing multiple types of cancer.

4. Rest, exhaustion, and physical activity: People who are undergoing treatment for cancer frequently experience extreme fatigue, sometimes known as fatigue. After the diagnosis has been made, the symptoms of exhaustion may also have a mental cause. The exhaustion that some individuals with breast cancer experience following treatment can linger for a significant amount of time, which can make it difficult for them to exercise and engage in other activities that they would like to do. Exercising, on the other hand, can help lessen feelings of exhaustion. The fact that patients who participate in an exercise program adapted to their specific requirements have improved physical and mental well-being and improved ability to deal with their condition is a crucial point to keep in mind.

It is typical for your fitness, endurance, and muscle strength to decrease if you are unwell and do not engage in a lot of physical activity while receiving treatment. Any strategy for physical activity ought to be tailored to your circumstances. A person who has never performed physical activity before cannot perform the same physical activity as someone who plays tennis twice a week. If it has been a few years since you last touched a piece of exercise equipment, you should begin carefully by going for short walks. You can also get more reviews on nutrition and physical activities from good evidence-based studies.

It is essential to talk with your healthcare team before starting anything. Get your physician's opinion about your exercise plans. The next step is finding a workout partner so you are not alone. A new exercise program can provide you with an additional boost of support to keep you going when the push isn't there. If you have family or friends involved in the program, they can provide you with extra support. It is okay to take a break whenever you need to do so. If you are fatigued, you must balance action and rest. Sometimes, it's hard for people to rest when they are used to working all day or caring for a household. Listen to your body and rest when you need to avoid burnout. Work or stressors can never finish.

Other helpful tips include;

- Learn enough about your breast cancer to make informed decisions about your care and treatment processes.
- Talking and keeping contact with other breast cancer patients and survivors
- Find someone to talk to about your feelings with diagnosis, treatment, and fears.
- Keep your friends and family close to prevent depression and isolation.
- Maintain close contact or intimacy with your partner.

Overdiagnosis and false positives are two diverse concepts in the context of breast cancer screening, and they differ in their implications and consequences.

1. False Positive results: False positives occur when a breast cancer screening test, such as a mammogram, suggests the presence of cancer when no cancer is present. False positives can be caused by various factors, including benign breast conditions, calcifications, cysts, or other non-cancerous abnormalities that can appear on a mammogram. False positives can lead to anxiety, additional testing, and sometimes unnecessary biopsies or surgical procedures. They are considered a downside of breast cancer screening, as they can cause emotional distress and increased healthcare costs.

2. Overdiagnosis: Overdiagnosis is the detection of breast cancers through screening that, if left undetected, would not have caused symptoms or harm during a person's lifetime. Overdiagnosis of breast cancer may result from the sensitivity of screening tests, which can identify very small or slow-growing cancers that might never progress to causing symptoms or harm. Some of these cancers are indolent and do not require treatment. It can lead to overtreatment, exposing individuals to the potential harms of cancer treatment (e.g., surgery, radiation, chemotherapy) when it may not be necessary. It can also result in unnecessary psychological and physical burdens for patients.

Necessary tools for Addressing False Positives and Overdiagnosis in breast cancer

1. Educate patients about the possibility of false positives and overdiagnosis in breast cancer screening. Encourage individuals to be informed about the screening process and its potential outcomes.

2. Promote shared decision-making between healthcare providers and patients. Discuss the benefits and risks of screening, allowing patients to make more personalized choices based on their individual risk factors and preferences.

3. Support ongoing research into more precise and targeted screening techniques that can reduce the occurrence of false positives and overdiagnosis while maintaining high sensitivity.

4. Implement comprehensive risk assessment tools to identify individuals at higher risk for breast cancer, enabling more tailored screening strategies.

5. Consider active surveillance for low-risk lesions found through screening rather than immediate aggressive treatment. This approach can help avoid overtreatment in cases of overdiagnosis.

6. Encourage individuals to seek a second opinion when facing a diagnosis or treatment decision based on screening results, especially if they are uncertain about the necessity of interventions.

7. Advocate for research and policies that prioritize reducing overdiagnosis and overtreatment while maintaining the benefits of early cancer detection.

8. Provide emotional and psychological support for individuals who experience false positives or overdiagnosis, as the associated stress and anxiety can be significant.
9. For those with indolent cancers, establish regular follow-up schedules to monitor their condition without immediately resorting to aggressive treatment.
10. Encourage healthcare professionals to stay updated with the latest guidelines and recommendations for breast cancer screening and diagnosis to provide their patients with the most current information and care.

Dealing with treatment choices for breast cancer

Breast Cancer is a malignancy developing in the breast tissues, typically in the lining epithelium of the milk ducts or in the lobules, which usually contain the milk-producing cells. Based on their origination region, they are known as ductal cancer if initiated in the milk ducts or lobular cancer if initiated in the lobules. Breast cancers are also categorized as hormone-negative or hormone-positive cancer, which is decided to depend upon their sensitivity to hormones like estrogen and progesterone.

The choices available for breast cancer treatment rely upon the type of breast cancer and the suggestion regarding staging. Staging is the course in which the spread of the disease and its progressive extent is demonstrated. Though it is the most common form of adenocarcinoma in women and is thought to be one of the fatal kinds of cancer, many progressive breast cancer treatment choices can help in remission for this disease if detected early in the course.

Once the diagnosis of cancer has been made, the doctors assess the pathology findings and create a plan that would be appropriate for the type of cancer and the stage to which the disease has advanced. Treatment approaches aim to plummet the spread of the disease, ultimately killing diseased cells and decreasing chances for future relapses. The doctors would pick a single or many treatment options depending on the patient's physical and medical conditions, which they may assess periodically. The **current** breast cancer treatment methods are generally classified as approved methods, which are still in clinical trials. Supported methods are those that are presently being practiced for causing remission in a multitude of breast cancer patients, while the methods still under clinical trials are those that are being tested for more competent results. The methods of breast cancer treatment comprise surgery, chemotherapy, hormone therapy, radiation treatments, and targeted treatment therapy.

What fundamental Misconception about tumor growth can do

Unfortunately, "malignant" tumors have been transformed into terrible monsters that have no other goal than to kill us as retribution for our sins or to abuse the body. This is due to fundamental misconceptions or a complete lack of knowledge about the reasons behind the growth of tumors. On the other hand, as you are going to discover, cancer is not working against us but rather in our favor. If we do not alter our understanding of what cancer is, it will continue to be resistant to therapy, particularly the most "advanced" approaches. If you are diagnosed with cancer, it is possible that cancer may not be a sickness but rather a component of the body's complex survival mechanisms.

It is suggested you are obligated to discover answers to the following critical questions:

i.   For what reasons does your body feel the need to produce cancer cells

against your will?

ii. Following the identification of these factors, is it possible for you to alter them? Which   factors determine the type of cancer that you have and the degree to which it has affected you?

iii. If cancer is a survival mechanism, what steps should be taken to prevent the body from   resorting to such extreme defense mechanisms?

iv. The body's basic genetic design constantly favors the preservation of life and protection   against adversities of any type; therefore, it is difficult to understand why the body would allow itself to destroy itself.

v. Do drastic treatments like radiation, chemotherapy, and surgery genuinely cure cancer, or do cancer patients who survive the disease recover for other reasons?

vi. In what ways do emotions such as anxiety, frustration, low self-worth, and repressed rage contribute to the development of cancer and its subsequent outcomes?

vii. Is there a spiritual development lesson that can be learned from cancer?

Finding answers that are both gratifying and practical to the problems raised above

is necessary to address the underlying causes of cancer. The Crucial Need for Answers to Improve Survival. Regardless of how far along the disease was, there has never been a person who has not been able to beat cancer. In the same way that there is a mechanism for the development of cancer, there must be a mechanism for the healing of cancer if even one individual has been successful in curing their disease. The capacity to do both is present in everyone on the globe. Even though you might not be able to change the diagnosis of cancer, you indeed can influence the damaging effects that the diagnosis may have on you. If you have been diagnosed with cancer, you may not be able to change the diagnosis. Two of the most influential factors that will determine whether or not you will be healthy in the future is how you perceive cancer and the actions you take after receiving a diagnosis of the disease.

Cancer has been transformed into a condition that has catastrophic effects for the majority of cancer patients and their families in today's society as a result of the widespread and dispassionate use of the term "cancer" to refer to a sickness that is a killer disease by both medical experts and the general public. The term "cancer" has come to be linked with extreme suffering, excruciating agony, and, ultimately, death.

It is of the utmost importance to be aware of the fact that, at this very minute, millions of people are walking around with malignancies concealed within their bodies without any knowledge that they have them. Similarly, millions of people miraculously recover from their cancers without ever being aware of it. If we want to avoid dying from cancer, the most critical question is not how advanced or terrible the cancer is; instead, it is what we need to do to prevent dying from it. Is it possible that some people can deal with cancer as if it were the flu? Are they simply fortunate, or does a system already in place cause the mending to occur? To put it another way, what is the factor that inhibits the body from naturally healing cancer, or what is the underlying factor that makes cancer so harmful, if it could be considered dangerous at all? It is not the degree of "viciousness" or the advanced stage that cancer appears to have progressed to that indicates the answers to all of these questions; instead, the answers lie with the response of the individual who is afflicted with the illness. Do you think that cancer may be classified as a disease? In the most likely scenario, you will respond with a "yes," One of the most critical questions, which is also one of the least frequently addressed, is "Why do you think cancer is a disease?" Because I am aware that cancer is responsible for the death of people daily. In addition, I would like to ask you the following question:

"How do you know that cancer is the cause of death for people?" If you were to argue that the majority of people who have cancer pass away, then it would be reasonable to assume that the illness itself is the cause of death. Furthermore, you can argue that all highly qualified medical professionals have told us this is the case. When you give a favorable response to your soul to ensure your survival, you will receive all of the answers you require, and this will be followed by healing and wellness through the adoption of a healthy way of life.

Recipes for supportive treatment of breast cancer

When it comes to treatment and recovery from cancer, it is necessary to strongly emphasize a well-balanced and nutritious diet, as this diet promotes overall health and supplies vital nutrients. Although it is essential to seek the advice of a healthcare practitioner or qualified dietician specializing in oncology, delicious and nutritious dishes can significantly assist cancer treatment and recovery. Supportive nutrition is essential for individuals undergoing breast cancer treatment. While a balanced diet cannot cure cancer, it can help maintain strength, support the immune system, and alleviate some treatment side effects.

Here are some suggested recipes that incorporate nutritious ingredients to aid in supportive treatment:

1. Ginger and Turmeric Smoothie: Ginger and turmeric are anti-inflammatory spices that can help reduce nausea and inflammation often associated with cancer treatment.

Ingredients:

1 cup Greek yogurt or dairy-free alternative

One ripe banana

1 tsp fresh grated ginger

1 tsp ground turmeric

1/2 tsp honey (optional)

a half cup of almond milk (or any other milk of your choice)

Put all of the ingredients into a blender, as directed in the instructions.

Blend until it is completely smooth.

If more milk is required to achieve the correct consistency, add it now.

Serve and take pleasure in it.

2. Vegetables and Quinoa: Quinoa is a grain that is high in protein and provides necessary nutrients. Vegetables, on the other hand, give a wide variety of vitamins and minerals that are crucial to one's general health.

Parts and pieces:

1 quart of quinoa

2 cups of water or broth made from vegetables

Two tablespoons of olive oil

One sliced onion of a small size

A total of two garlic cloves, minced

florets of broccoli and one cup

1 cup of sliced bell peppers consisting of a variety of colors

One teaspoonful of chopped mushrooms

Peas, one cup's worth

Tomato sauce or low-sodium soy sauce, two tablespoons

One teaspoon of freshly grated ginger

You can modify the amount of red pepper flakes to your liking.

To taste, season with salt and pepper

Follow these instructions to rinse the quinoa properly in a sieve with fine mesh. The quinoa should be combined with either water or vegetable broth in a saucepan. Bring to a boil, immediately reduce the heat to low, cover, and continue to simmer for around fifteen minutes or until the quinoa is cooked.

Olive oil should be heated in a big skillet or wok over medium-high heat throughout the quinoa cooking. Sauté the onion and garlic until they release their sweet aroma. The snow peas, bell peppers, mushrooms, and broccoli should be added to the skillet. Cook the vegetables in a stir-fry until they are crisp-tender.Mix the ingredients in a small bowl: grated ginger, red pepper flakes, soy sauce or tamari, salt, and pepper.

Add the sauce to the stir-fried vegetables, then simmer for two to three minutes.To finish, sprinkle the stir-fried vegetables with fresh herbs such as cilantro or parsley and serve them on top of the quinoa that has been cooked.

3. Creamy Tomato Soup: This comforting soup provides hydration and essential nutrients, making it suitable for individuals experiencing treatment side effects.

Ingredients:

- One can (28 oz) diced tomatoes
- One small onion, chopped
- Two cloves garlic, minced
- 1 cup low-sodium vegetable broth
- 1/2 cup unsweetened almond milk (or dairy-free milk of choice)
- 1 tsp olive oil
- 1/2 tsp dried basil
- 1/2 tsp dried oregano

- Salt and pepper to taste
- Fresh basil leaves (for garnish, optional)

Instructions:

In a large pot, heat the olive oil over medium heat. Add chopped onions and garlic. Sauté until onions are translucent.

Add diced tomatoes (with juice), vegetable broth, dried basil, dried oregano, salt, and pepper. Bring the mixture to a boil, then reduce the heat and simmer for about 10 minutes. Blend the soup with an immersion or a countertop blender until smooth. Return the blended soup to the pot, add almond milk, and heat through. Serve hot, garnished with fresh basil leaves if desired.

Exercise recommendations for breast cancer survivors

Exercise can be a valuable supportive treatment for breast cancer patients and survivors. It can help improve physical and emotional well-being, reduce treatment side effects, and enhance overall quality of life. Here are some exercise recommendations for individuals affected by breast cancer:

1. **Consult Your Healthcare Team:** Before starting any exercise program, consult your healthcare team, including your oncologist and a qualified physical therapist or certified cancer exercise specialist. They can provide personalized guidance based on your condition, treatment plan, and potential limitations.
2. **Aerobic Exercise:** Aerobic or cardiovascular exercises, such as walking, jogging, swimming, or cycling, can help improve cardiovascular fitness, boost energy levels, and manage treatment-related fatigue. Start with gentle,

low-impact activities and gradually increase intensity as you build stamina. Aim for at least 150 minutes of moderate-intensity aerobic exercise per week, as the American Cancer Society recommends.

3. **Strength Training:** Strength training exercises using resistance bands, dumbbells, or body weight can help maintain muscle mass and strength, which may be affected by cancer treatments. Focus on all major muscle groups, including the arms, legs, chest, back, and core. Begin with light weights and progress slowly under the guidance of a fitness professional.

4. **Flexibility and Stretching:** Stretching exercises can improve flexibility, reduce muscle tightness, and enhance joint mobility. Incorporate gentle stretching routines into your exercise regimen to help prevent muscle stiffness and joint discomfort. Yoga and tai chi are excellent options that combine stretching with relaxation and mindfulness.

5. **Balance and Coordination:** Balance and coordination exercises can reduce the risk of falls and improve overall stability. Activities like Pilates, balance drills, and functional movements can be beneficial.

6. **Mindful Movement Practices:** Mind-body practices like yoga and meditation can reduce stress and anxiety, improve sleep quality, and enhance emotional well-being. These practices can help you connect with your body and promote relaxation.

7. **Hydration and Rest:** Stay well-hydrated before, during, and after exercise, especially if you're experiencing treatment-related side effects like nausea or diarrhea. Listen to your body and rest when needed. Fatigue is common during cancer treatment, so it's essential to prioritize rest and recovery.

8. **Safety Precautions:** Pay attention to any side effects or discomfort during exercise, and communicate these to your healthcare team. Wear

comfortable clothing and supportive shoes. Exercises with a high impact should be avoided because they can increase the likelihood of injuries or stress fractures.

9. Make Gradual Progress: Begin your workout regimen cautiously and gradually raise both the duration and the intensity of your workout program. Be patient with yourself and set realistic goals.

10. **Community and Support:** Consider joining a cancer-specific exercise class or support group to connect with others going through a similar journey. It can provide motivation and a sense of community.

Examples of exercise for breast cancer patients

Exercise can be an essential component of breast cancer recovery and overall well-being. Below are some examples of exercises that can be beneficial for individuals recovering from breast cancer surgery, particularly those who have had mastectomies or lumpectomies. These exercises should be done under the guidance of a healthcare professional or physical therapist to ensure they are safe and suitable for your specific situation.

1. **Arm Circles:**
    i. Stand or sit up straight with your feet shoulder-width apart.
    ii. Extend your arms straight out to the sides.
    iii. Make small circles with your arms, gradually increasing the size of the circles.

    iv. Repeat for 10-15 circles in each direction.

2. **Wall Angels:**
   i. Stand with your back against a wall, feet hip-width apart.
   ii. Keep your arms relaxed by your sides.
   iii. Slowly raise your arms overhead, maintaining contact with the wall.
   iv. Lower your arms back down to your sides.
   v. Repeat for 10-15 repetitions.

3. **Pendulum Swing:**
   i. Stand next to a sturdy surface like a table or chair, placing one hand on it for support.
   ii. Bend forward slightly at the hips.
   iii. Let your affected arm hang down and relax.
   iv. Gently swing your arm forward and backward, then side to side, and finally, in a circular motion.
   v. Perform these swings for 1-2 minutes in each direction.

4. **Scapular Retraction:**
   i. Sit or stand with your arms relaxed by your sides.
   ii. Squeeze your shoulder blades together by pulling them towards each other.
   iii. Hold for a few seconds, then release.
   iv. Repeat for 10-15 repetitions.

5. **Arm Raises:**
   i. Stand or sit with your back straight.
   ii. Hold a small weight or a water bottle in your hand.
   iii. Slowly raise your affected arm out to the side and overhead.
   iv. Lower your arm back down to your side.
   v. Repeat for 10-15 repetitions.

6. **Chest Stretch:**
   i. Stand with your feet shoulder-width apart.

ii. Clasp your hands behind your back.

iii. Gently pull your arms backward to open up your chest.

iv. Hold for 20-30 seconds, feeling the stretch in your chest and shoulders.

7. **Breathing Exercises:**

    i. Deep breathing exercises can help improve lung capacity and overall well-being.

    ii. Sit comfortably and take slow, deep breaths through your nose, expanding your chest and diaphragm.

    iii. Exhale slowly through your mouth.

    iv. Repeat this deep breathing pattern for several minutes.

8. **Yoga and Tai Chi:**

    i. These mind-body practices can help improve flexibility, balance, and overall well-being. Look for classes designed for breast cancer survivors, which offer modifications and support.

Perfect foods against breast cancer

One of the most critical factors in promoting general health and lowering the risk of breast cancer is eating a well-balanced diet that is rich in nutrients. There is, indeed, no one meal that may prevent or cure breast cancer; nevertheless, a diet that is abundant in certain nutrients and foods may help reduce the risk of developing breast cancer and maintain breast health. Here are some foods and nutrients that are considered beneficial in the fight against breast cancer:

1. **Cruciferous Vegetables:**

   i.   Broccoli, cauliflower, Brussels sprouts, kale, and cabbage contain compounds like sulforaphane and indole-3-carbinol, which may have cancer-fighting properties.

   ii.   Incorporate these vegetables into your diet through stir-fries, salads, or steamed side dishes.

2. **Berries:**

   i.   Blueberries, strawberries, raspberries, and blackberries are rich in antioxidants, including anthocyanins and ellagic acid, associated with reduced cancer risk.

   ii.   Enjoy berries as a snack, in smoothies, or as a topping for yogurt or oatmeal.

3. **Fatty Fish:**

   i.   Fatty fish like salmon, mackerel, and sardines are high in omega-3 fatty acids, which have anti-inflammatory properties and may help reduce the risk of breast cancer.

   ii.   Aim for at least two servings of fatty fish per week.

4. **Turmeric and Curcumin:**

   i.   Turmeric contains curcumin, a compound with potent anti-inflammatory and antioxidant properties.

   ii.   Add turmeric to curries, soups, or smoothies.

5. **Leafy Greens:**

   i.   Spinach, Swiss chard, and other leafy greens are rich in vitamins, minerals, and antioxidants that support overall health.

   ii.   Incorporate them into salads, sandwiches, or sautéed dishes.

6. **Flaxseeds:**

i. Flaxseeds are an excellent source of lignans, which are phytoestrogens that have the potential to offer a preventive impact against breast cancer that is caused by hormone deficiencies.
ii. Ground flaxseeds can be sprinkled on cereal or yogurt or used in baking.

7. **Green Tea:**
   i. Green tea contains polyphenols, particularly epigallocatechin gallate (EGCG), which has antioxidant and anti-inflammatory properties.
   ii. Enjoy green tea as a beverage, or use it as a smoothie base.

8. **Garlic and Onions:**
   i. Garlic and onions contain organosulfur compounds that may help reduce the risk of breast cancer.
   ii. Use them in cooking to add flavor and health benefits to your meals.

9. **Tomatoes:**
   i. Tomatoes are a good source of lycopene, an antioxidant that may lower the risk of breast cancer.
   ii. Incorporate tomatoes into salads, sauces, or sandwiches.

10. **Nuts and Seeds:**
    i. Almonds, walnuts, and sunflower seeds are rich in nutrients, including vitamin E and healthy fats, which support overall health.
    ii. Enjoy a handful of unsalted nuts and seeds as a snack.

11. **Whole Grains:**
    i. Whole grains like brown rice, quinoa, and whole wheat contain fiber and essential nutrients that promote overall health.
    ii. Choose whole grains over refined grains for improved nutrition.

12. **Low-Fat Dairy or Dairy Alternatives:**

Foods that are low in fat or dairy alternatives fortified with calcium and vitamin D can assist in maintaining strong bones, hence lowering the chance of developing breast cancer.

Here are some other foods that are great for preventing cancer.

Apples (fruit)

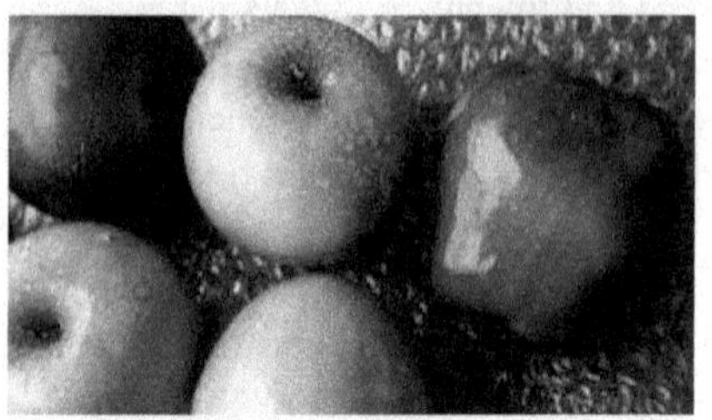

Regarding health, the proverb "an apple a day keeps the doctor away" rings almost entirely true. Apples are a source of polyphenols, which have been shown to possess anticancer characteristics. There is some evidence that polyphenols derived from plants can reduce inflammation, cardiovascular disease, and infections. Polyphenols have been shown to have anticancer and tumor-fighting capabilities, according to specific research. One example is the polyphenol phloretin, which can inhibit a protein known as glucose transporter 2 (GLUT2). This protein is involved in the progression of some types of cancer to more advanced stages of cell growth.

Toasted tomatoes

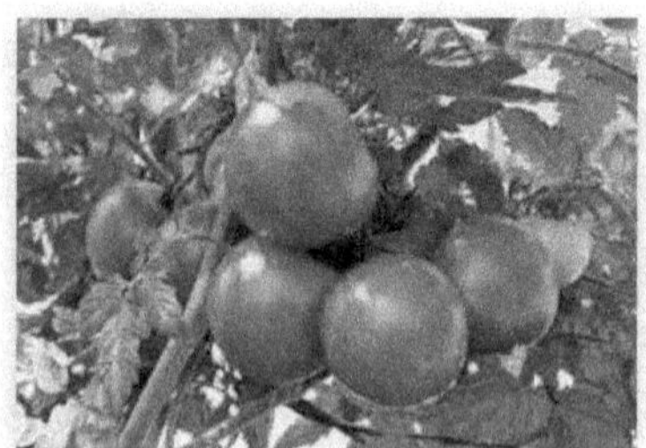

Not only are tomatoes delicious, but they are also quite healthful. Because of their many positive effects on health, tomatoes ought to be a regular part of every person's diet. In Better Homes and Gardens, the cancer-fighting advantages of tomatoes are described as follows: "This fruit or vegetable is the very definition of a superfood that can help fight cancer. In addition to containing lycopene, an antioxidant phytochemical that aids in the prevention of cardiovascular disease, tomatoes are also an excellent source of vitamins A, C, and E, which are all known to be antagonists of free radicals that are beneficial to the development of cancer. On top of the pizza dough that has already been prepared, tomatoes, spinach, and peppers are layered, and then tomato sauce and mozzarella with part-skim cheese are added. Add some cherry tomatoes to the salad that you are making with romaine lettuce. Using sliced tomatoes, lettuce, and either shredded broccoli or alfalfa sprouts, stuff your sandwiches with delicious ingredients. You should find a method to incorporate tomatoes into your diet daily.

carrots (carrots)

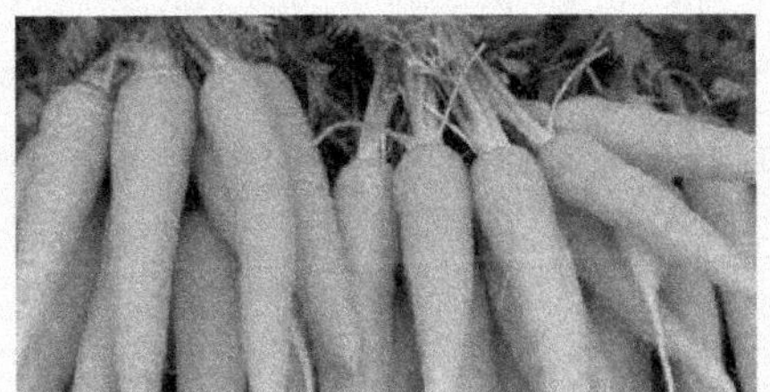

Carrots are a good source of several essential nutrients, such as vitamins K and A and antioxidants.

Additionally, carrots have a significantly high concentration of beta-carotene, the pigment that gives them their distinctive orange color. According to findings from recent research, beta-carotene is an essential component in bolstering the immune system and may also be able to prevent some types of cancer. Beta-carotene has been linked to a reduction in the incidence of breast and prostate cancer, according to an analysis of eight research that was conducted on the subject.

Fish that are high in fat

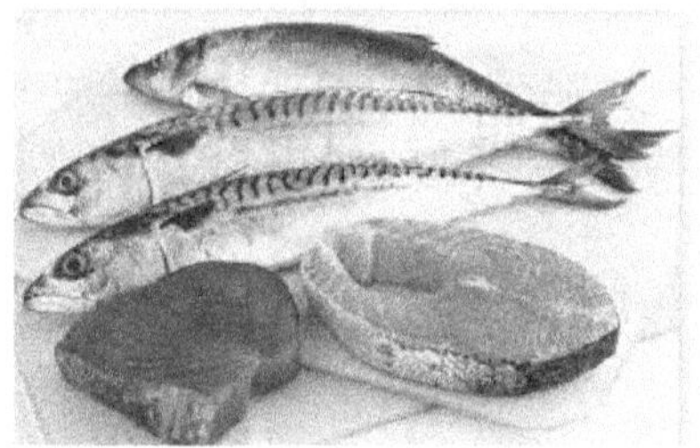

Among the essential nutrients that can be found in abundance in fatty fish, such as salmon, mackerel, and anchovies, are vitamin B, potassium, and omega-3 fatty acids. Compared to those whose diets were low in freshwater fish, those containing a significant amount of freshwater fish had a lower chance of developing colorectal cancer.

The kale

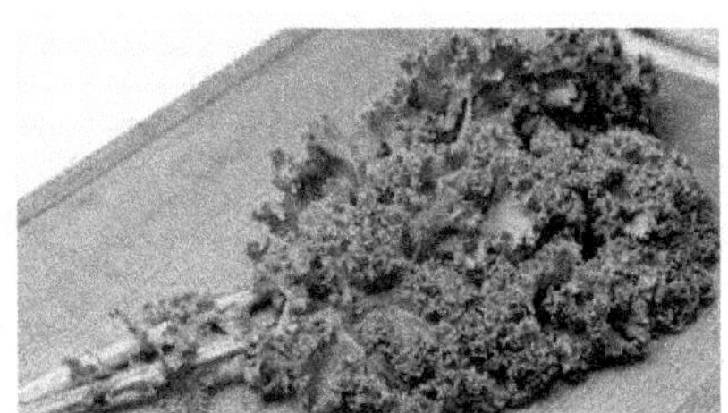

In the world of cooking, kale is in the spotlight right now. Your body can maintain its health, receive the nutrients it needs, and battle cancer with its assistance. Kale is another type of cruciferous vegetable with a high concentration of vitamin C and vitamin K. These vitamins are known to be effective in preventing cancers such as breast, lung, prostate, and colon cancer.

cabbage (cabbage)

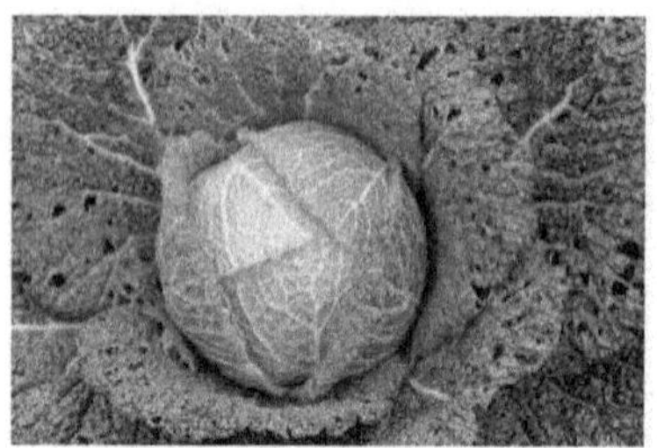

Although it is a core ingredient in many different ethnic cuisines, cabbage may not be as commonly used in other cuisines. In contrast, it aids in the prevention of cancer in our bodies. Breast cancer, colon cancer, and rectal cancer are all reduced in risk when cabbage is consumed. Consuming it in its raw form or with only a tiny amount of cooking is recommended to benefit fully from its cancer-fighting effects.

Legumes (plural)

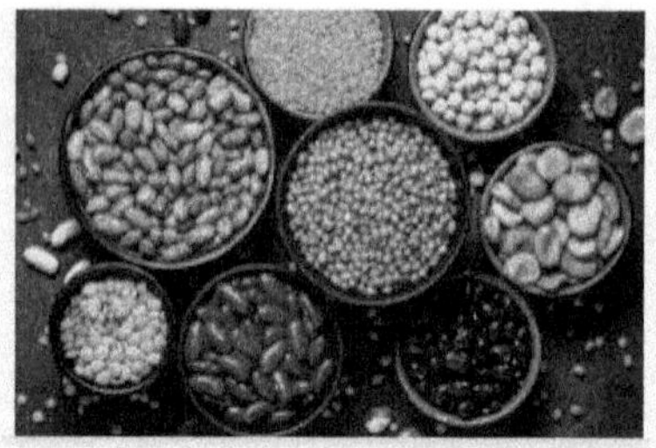

As a result of their high fiber content, legumes, which include beans, peas, and lentils, can potentially reduce the likelihood of an individual developing cancer.

Grilled salmon with quinoa and roasted veggies are examples of meals that are high in protein. Baked chicken breast served with brown rice and broccoli that has been cooked. Soup made with lentils and toast made with nutritious grains.

Roasted vegetables, such as carrots, bell peppers, and Brussels sprouts seasoned with herbs and olive oil, are examples of meals that are exceptionally rich in antioxidants. Coconut milk, banana, spinach, and kale are the ingredients in this green smoothie.

Immune-enhancing foods include chicken soup with ginger and turmeric, accompanied with veggies. Whole wheat spaghetti and spinach accompanied by prawns that have been sautéed with garlic and lemon. Flaxseeds and Greek yogurt, topped with a variety of berries and a mix of them. Some foods high in nutrients include hummus with carrots and cucumber sticks. Almonds that have been cut and Greek yogurt that has been drizzled with honey. Dates, nuts, and seeds are mixed to create energy balls.

Drinks that are hydrating include water that has been infused with cucumber, lemon, and mint. Green tea with a bit of honey added to it. Lime juices that have been freshly squeezed. Please keep in mind that the purpose of these recipes is not to substitute for the individualized dietary recommendations provided by medical specialists. It is essential to consider any nutritional limitations or special requirements that may differ for each individual, as these may change depending on the type and stage of cancer and the treatments being followed.

Conquering your Fear

Breast cancer patients should not be allowed any room at all to be afraid because fear is one of the significant elements that lead to the mortality of breast cancer patients. The primary concern should be how to recharge your mental batteries and revalue your self-worth, how to let go of bad energy and welcome positive transformation in your life, how to reconnect with your unique talents and turn roadblocks into building blocks, how to reframe the vision of who you want to be and how you want to project yourself, how to reclaim the person you are destined to be and the life you want to live without fear, and how to reclaim the life you want to live. It is important to note that conquering fear is a gradual process, and it's okay to seek professional help or rely on your support system when needed. You are not alone on this Journey, and there is hope, strength, and resilience within you to face breast cancer with courage and determination.

Conquering fear as a breast cancer patient is a formidable challenge, but it's essential for your well-being and recovery. Here are some strategies to help you navigate this problematic Journey:

1. **Knowledge is Power:** Educate yourself about breast cancer, including the type and stage of your cancer, treatment options, and potential side effects. Understanding your condition can help demystify it and reduce fear.
2. **Consult a Healthcare Team:** Build a supportive healthcare team of oncologists, surgeons, nurses, and support staff. Discuss your concerns, treatment plan, and expected outcomes with them. Having a trusted team can alleviate anxiety.

3. **Support System:** Lean on friends and family for emotional support. Consider joining a breast cancer support group to connect with others who have experienced similar challenges.

4. **Mindfulness and Meditation:** Practice mindfulness and meditation techniques help to manage anxiety and stress. These techniques can help you stay grounded and focused on the present moment.

5. **Ask Questions:** Don't hesitate to ask questions and seek clarification from your healthcare team. Understanding your treatment options, potential side effects, and prognosis can reduce uncertainty.

6. **Set Realistic Expectations:** Recognize that the cancer journey may have ups and downs. Set realistic expectations for yourself and understand that recovery may take time.

7. Support on an emotional level: Think about having a conversation with a therapist or counselor who specializes in dealing with concerns associated with cancer. They can aid your ability to deal with fear, worry, and the emotional toll that illness takes.

8. Pay attention to good nutrition, regular exercise, and sufficient sleep to maintain a healthy lifestyle. A healthy body tolerates treatment more efficiently, contributing to overall well-being.

9. Decision-Making Regarding Treatment: Be an active participant in the decision-making process regarding your treatment plan. Talk with your healthcare team about the benefits and drawbacks of each alternative, and then select the strategy that best fits your priorities and objectives.

10. **Express Your Feelings:** Expressing your fears and concerns to your loved ones or support group is okay. Sharing your feelings can be therapeutic and help you process your emotions.

11. Stay informed about advancements in breast cancer treatment and support services. Knowledge about available resources can provide hope and empowerment.

12. **Visualization:** Practice visualization techniques where you imagine positive outcomes and envision yourself overcoming challenges. This visualization can help reduce fear and increase optimism.

13. **Celebrate Small Victories:** Acknowledge and celebrate small achievements and milestones during your treatment journey. These victories can boost your confidence and morale.

14. Exhibit self-compassion by treating yourself with kindness: Be conscious that fear is a normal reaction to a cancer diagnosis. Permit yourself to experience your feelings without passing judgment on them.

15. **Plan for the Future:** Consider long-term plans like life after cancer treatment. Setting goals and looking forward to the future can provide hope and motivation.

Post-treatment complications associated with breast cancer.

The Post-treatment symptoms/conditions associated with breast cancer are as follows;

1. **Neuropathy**: The hands and feet are often affected by neuropathy, which is a form of discomfort that is brought on by damage to the nerves. Neuropathy is most commonly seen following chemotherapy. This illness can manifest itself in various ways, including numbness or pain, heightened sensitivity to hot or cold temperatures, or weakening of the muscles of the hands and feet. On the other hand, the symptoms disappear for some individuals once the treatment is finished. On the other hand, it may be severe for specific people and may not disappear entirely.

2. Thinning hair or hair loss, also known as **alopecia**, can occur with certain types of chemo- and radiation therapy and hormonal, targeted, or immune therapies. For many, hair loss is temporary. But, whether mild or severe, it can be traumatic, especially for women. To prepare, talk to your doctor about if, when, and to what degree your treatment strategy can cause hair loss and if there are options to potentially stave off loss, like cold capping (scalp hypothermia).

3. **Lymphedema**—an abnormal swelling in the arms, underarms, hands, breast, chest, or back—is a side effect of breast cancer surgery and radiation treatment. When lymph nodes are removed or damaged during these procedures, the lymph (clear fluid that circulates the body to remove substances from tissues) cannot circulate properly and builds up.

4. Other unwanted side effects that survivors may experience include **sexual dysfunction, changes in libido, early menopause, and vaginal discomfort**. Sexual health is an essential aspect of survivorship, and these symptoms are nothing to be embarrassed about. If you're experiencing any of them, talk to your breast cancer care team.

Prevailing over the diagnosis cum treatment of breast cancer and answering a survivor

A breast cancer patient is termed a survivor after having no signs of *cancer* after finishing treatment. · Living with, through, and beyond cancer can also make a breast cancer patient be referred to as a breast cancer survivor. Breast cancer survivorship is more than just surviving cancer. It includes your long-term physical, mental, emotional, and financial health. Most commonly, the survivorship phase is thought to start after completing active treatment with surgery, chemotherapy, or radiation therapy, if needed. Although different categories of survivorship may not be explored here, the mental readiness to live life to the fullest to prevent post-treatment complications and live a long, satisfying, and happy life after treatment is over.

Prevailing over a breast cancer diagnosis and treatment is a challenging and courageous journey.

Here are some essential steps and strategies to help you navigate this complex path:

i. **Accept Your Emotions:** It's completely normal to experience a wide range of emotions, including fear, anger, sadness, and uncertainty, upon receiving a breast cancer diagnosis. Allow yourself to feel these emotions and give yourself permission to grieve and process your feelings.

ii. **Gather a Support System:** Contact your friends and family for emotional support. Consider joining a breast cancer support group to connect with others who have faced similar challenges. Having a solid support system can provide comfort and understanding.

iii. **Educate Yourself:** Seek information about your specific type and stage of breast cancer, treatment options, and potential side effects. Understanding your condition and treatment plan can empower you to make informed decisions.

iv. **Communicate with Your Healthcare Team:** Build a trusting relationship with your healthcare providers, including oncologists, surgeons, and nurses. Ask questions, express your concerns, and actively participate in discussions about your treatment plan.

v. **Treatment Decision-Making:** Collaborate with your healthcare team to make treatment decisions that align with your goals and values. Consider seeking a second opinion if you have doubts or want to explore different treatment options.

vi. **Maintain a Healthy Lifestyle:** Focus on proper nutrition, regular exercise, and adequate rest. A healthy lifestyle can improve your physical and emotional well-being and support your body during treatment.

vii. **Mind-Body Practices:** Explore mindfulness meditation, relaxation techniques, or yoga to manage stress and anxiety. These practices can help you stay grounded and cope with the emotional challenges of cancer.

viii. **Advocate for Yourself:** Be your advocate in your healthcare journey. Keep detailed records of your medical history, treatment plans, and medications. Feel free to ask for clarification or express your needs and concerns.

ix. **Supportive Therapies:** Consider complementary therapies like acupuncture, massage, or art therapy to enhance your well-being during treatment.

x. **Positive Visualization:** Practice positive visualization and affirmations. Visualize yourself healing, gaining strength, and overcoming challenges on your path to recovery.

xi. **Celebrate Small Victories:** Acknowledge and celebrate every milestone, no matter how small it may seem. Each step forward is a victory on your Journey to becoming a survivor.

xii. **Set Future Goals:** Plan for life after treatment. Set personal goals and aspirations to look forward to, providing motivation and hope for the future.

xiii. **Regular Follow-Up Care:** After treatment, you must continue with regular follow-up appointments and screenings to monitor your health. Staying vigilant about your post-treatment care is vital for long-term well-being.

xiv. **Embrace Survivorship:** As you progress through treatment and recovery, embrace the identity of a cancer survivor. Share your story to inspire others and support those facing similar challenges.

The arduous Journey of beast cancer survivorship

Becoming a breast cancer survivor is a testament to the strength and resilience that resides within every individual facing this challenging diagnosis. It is a journey marked by courage, determination, and unwavering hope. While the road may be arduous, the transformation from a breast cancer patient to a survivor is a remarkable story of triumph over adversity. This Journey is a source of inspiration, offering valuable lessons in resilience, self-discovery, and the power of the human spirit. Becoming a breast cancer survivor is a testament to your strength and resilience.

While the Journey may be challenging, you have the inner resources and support to prevail over this diagnosis and treatment. Stay focused on your healing, and remember that you are not alone in your fight against breast cancer.

The Diagnosis: The Journey to becoming a breast cancer survivor begins with a diagnosis that can shake the very foundation of one's life if not properly guided. Hearing those words, "You have breast cancer," can be an overwhelming and emotional experience. It marks the beginning of a path filled with uncertainty and fear. It is a moment that forces individuals to confront their mortality and face the daunting challenges that lie ahead.

The Initial Fear: Fear is an ever-present companion on the Journey to survivorship. The fear of the unknown, the fear of treatment, and the fear of what the future holds can be paralyzing. It is expected to experience a whirlwind of emotions, including anxiety, sadness, anger, and doubt. These emotions are a natural response to the profound disruption that cancer brings to one's life.

Seeking Support: One of the critical turning points on the path to survivorship is seeking support. Whether from family, friends, or a community of fellow survivors, support plays an integral role in navigating the challenges of cancer.

Sharing experiences, seeking guidance, and finding solace in the company of others who have faced similar journeys can provide comfort and encouragement.

The Treatment Journey: The treatment journey is a formidable and often grueling aspect of the battle against breast cancer. It may include surgeries, chemotherapy, radiation therapy, and various medications.

Each step in the treatment process presents its own set of physical and emotional challenges. The side effects, the physical toll, and the uncertainty of how one's body will respond can be daunting.

Strength and Resilience: Becoming a breast cancer survivor requires unwavering strength and resilience. It is about facing each treatment session with determination and gracefully enduring the difficult days. Survivorship is a testament to the tenacity of the human spirit, the ability to endure hardships, and the refusal to surrender to adversity.

Support System: Throughout the Journey, a support system becomes a lifeline. Family and friends' love, care, and encouragement provide an anchor during turbulent times. The dedication and expertise of healthcare professionals become invaluable guides on the path to healing. Support groups and networks of fellow survivors offer a sense of belonging and shared understanding.

Hope and Healing: Hope drives the transformation from a breast cancer patient to a survivor. It is the belief that a brighter future awaits and that healing is possible. Hope empowers individuals to push forward, even when the road seems impossible. It is a beacon of light that dispels the darkness of fear and uncertainty.

Celebrating Survivorship: The Journey to becoming a breast cancer survivor is punctuated by big and small milestones. Celebrating these victories—clear scans, the completion of treatment, and the return to a sense of normalcy—becomes a source of joy and gratitude. It is a testament to the power of resilience and the triumph of the human spirit.

Challenges Breast Cancer Survivors May Face

If you've completed treatment for breast cancer, you may think that the hard part is over once you've completed treatment, but you may face new challenges that come with survivorship. Some of these challenges include;

Reduced Number of Requests for Medical Care: Patients who have survived breast cancer are accustomed to being under the continual supervision of a care team while adhering to a comprehensive care plan while they are undergoing treatment. Following therapy, you could experience feelings of being on your own, without a plan, and wondering what to do next.

There are new feelings, including guilt: The realization that their treatment and diagnosis could have been worse is something that frequently strikes breast cancer survivors, and this realization can lead to feelings of guilt.

Survivors may also experience feelings of guilt if they do not immediately experience happiness, even though they have been looking forward to the conclusion of treatment. Survivors may also experience anxiety about returning to their previous jobs or schools, as well as the responsibility of taking care of their families. They can still experience a great deal of fatigue. Another possibility is that they will exhibit symptoms of anxiety or depression.

Image of the Body: The treatment for breast cancer may include significant alterations to the body, such as surgical removal of both breasts (bilateral) or only one breast (unilateral). There is also the possibility that survivors have undergone a lumpectomy or surgery to remove a tumor from their breast, which might result in a change in the shape of the breast. In addition, the cancer treatment may cause some cancer drugs to promote weight gain. One more issue that some people have trouble with is how their hair grows back after chemotherapy; it may be thicker, thinner, curlier, or even a different color overall. Hair loss and regeneration can significantly influence the viewpoint of survivors and their capacity to feel like themselves again.

Peace of Mind Awareness Screening: Individuals who have undergone a mastectomy do not need to get annual screening mammography because the breast tissue has been removed. This is because it is widespread for individuals to overanalyze every symptom or worry that they are not receiving sufficient screening for the recurrence of cancer.

Additional Health Concerns: As a result of their treatment for breast cancer, survivors frequently encounter a variety of health issues, including but not limited to pain, exhaustion, sexual dysfunction, dermatological concerns, cardiovascular issues, low bone density, and other health issues. During chemotherapy, they may even encounter cognitive problems, such as mental fogginess, difficulty concentrating, and difficulty juggling multiple tasks at once. This syndrome is frequently called "chemo-brain" and typically gets better over time.

Dealing With Breast Cancer Survivorship Challenges

With all these challenges in mind, here are a few tips for embracing your new normal after surviving breast cancer. Establish Primary Care: One of the most essential things survivors can do after breast cancer treatment is to make sure they have a primary care clinician. They are an integral part of the team that helps manage survivorship issues and essential health maintenance. A primary care clinician can also facilitate a referral to a mental health professional if needed. Suppose survivors have access to a survivorship program. In that case, they can work with their care team to create a survivorship care plan, which includes a plan for surveillance and general health maintenance, including screening for other cancers and chronic health conditions. It also provides resources for seeking more information and assistance after receiving a breast cancer diagnosis and undergoing treatment. Sharing as much personal and health information as possible with your primary care clinician is essential to bridge the initial gap between your cancer treatment and continued primary care.

Be Patient: Even after treatment, your physical body and emotional spirit still heal. It's important to remember that fatigue and other side effects of treatment don't go away as soon as treatment ends. Whether it was surgery, radiation therapy, chemotherapy, or all of the above, a survivor's body just went through a significant trauma and needs time to heal. Medications may be necessary to prevent cancer from returning and can also have side effects that impact quality of life. So wear patience as a cloth.

Embrace a Healthier Lifestyle: Some people equate surviving cancer with getting a new lease on life. It's an excellent opportunity to Eschew bad habits and focus on things that make them feel good — inside and out. Eating a heart-healthy diet high in antioxidants is one of the best and easiest ways to boost your health. Certain foods can strengthen your immune system and help you maintain healthy body weight, which are primary factors in the fight against cancer. Some of these foods include broccoli, tomatoes, blueberries, and walnuts . Exercise can also play a massive role in helping you feel energized again. Evidence shows that exercise boosts your mood and memory and can even help reverse the effects of stress. Exercise can also help with bone health, reducing the risk of osteoporosis.

Choose How You Move On: "Breast cancer doesn't have to be a survivor's identity," "It's a health condition they need to manage or have managed, but it doesn't have to define who they are."Everyone will handle survivorship differently, so survivors should not compare themselves to others.

Look to the Future: Life after breast cancer will have its ups and downs. Some days will be better than others, but survivors will always have a unique perspective on life to draw from. All of the feelings and concerns that come with survivorship are entirely normal. With patience, support from friends and family, and frequent checkups with their healthcare providers, they can gradually find a new normal.

Using workouts and simple lifestyle changes to prevent occurrence and recurrence.
Exercise strengthens your heart and improves your circulation. The **increased blood flow raises the oxygen levels in your body**. Exercise helps lower your risk of heart diseases such as high cholesterol, coronary artery disease, and heart attack. Regular exercise can also lower your blood pressure and triglyceride levels.

When it comes to the many aspects of lifestyle, physical exercise has the most significant impact on the outcomes of breast cancer. After receiving a diagnosis of breast cancer, a rise in body weight of more than ten percent is associated with an increased risk of death from breast cancer as well as death from any cause. On the other hand, there are valid reasons to discourage even moderate weight gain due to its detrimental consequences on one's mood and perception of their body. There is a correlation between being overweight or obese and having a lower chance of survival for women.

On the other hand, women who engage in moderate exercise, which consists of thirty minutes of physical activity five days per week or seventy-five minutes of intensive exercise per week, had a much lower risk of breast cancer recurrence and breast cancer death.

On the other hand, it does not appear that diet has any influence on the recurrence of breast cancer. Some beneficial approaches to lower your risk of occurrence and recurrence include maintaining a healthy diet, engaging in physical activity, and practicing mindful mental health.

Exploring the options for preventing the occurrence and recurrence of breast cancer

1. Maintain A Healthy Weight by fitting physical activity and movement into your life each day, Limiting time in front of the TV and computer, trying to stand more, and Consuming a diet that is abundant in fruits, vegetables, and grains that are whole, and Choose smaller quantities, eat more slowly, and reduce the amount of sugary beverages you consume.

2. Get some exercise Regularly by selecting activities that you enjoy, such as walking, gardening, and dancing; make exercise a habit by setting aside the same amount of time for it each day; go to the gym during lunchtime or take a walk after dinner; keep it fun and stay motivated by exercising with someone else; and be active as a family by going to the park, taking walks, and playing active games.

3. Refrain from smoking

4. Consume a Healthy Diet. Include fruits and vegetables in every meal that you eat. Add some fruit to your bowl of cereal. As a snack, consume some vegetables. Instead of red and processed meat, choose chicken, fish, or beans as your protein source. Opt for cereal made with whole grains and bread made with whole wheat rather than sugar and white bread. Opt for recipes prepared with olive or canola oil, as these oils contain a wealth of beneficial fats. Reduce your consumption of fast food and snacks purchased from stores (such as cookies). A balanced diet is essential; if you consistently fall short, consider taking a regular multivitamin.

5. Reduce the amount of alcohol you consume; zero may be the best option. During meals and parties, select beverages that do not include alcohol. It is best to steer clear of events that involve drinking. If you believe you have a problem with alcohol, you should consult with a healthcare expert. Talk to youngsters about the risks associated with alcohol and drugs when the situation calls for it. You should take precautions against the sun and stay away from tanning beds.The 10 a.m. to 4 p.m., considered peak burning hours, should be avoided at all costs.

6.To protect oneself, this is the most effective method. Helmets, long-sleeved shirts, and sunscreens with an SPF of 30 or higher are recommended. Avoid using tanning beds or tanning booths at any cost. Protect children first, and always wear sunscreen and appropriate attire.

7. Take precautions to avoid contracting sexually transmitted diseases. Viral infections that are spread by sexual contact, such as human papillomavirus (HPV), hepatitis, and HIV, have the potential to cause a variety of malignancies. The risk can be reduced by taking precautions against certain illnesses.

Always make an effort to engage in safer sexual practices since this will reduce the likelihood of contracting a sexually transmitted infection.

8. Participate in screening examinations. Various essential screening tests are available, each of which can contribute to cancer prevention. While some of these tests can detect cancer at an earlier stage, when it is more amenable to treatment, others can assist in preventing cancer from occurring in the first place.

Say goodbye and beat your cancer scare forever.
Putting fear in a corner is one of the ways of saying goodbye to cancer and also a way to avoid the different fears from diagnosis, treatment, and post-treatment stages, which is a key to survivorship. The fear of cancer returning. I'm clean now, but my mind doesn't dare believe it should all be quiet. Instead, do the following;

- Look optimistically to the future
- Staying away from tobacco.
- Protect your skin from overexposure to ultraviolet rays from the sun and tanning beds.
- I am eating lots of fruits and vegetables.
- I am keeping a healthy weight.
- Be physically active.
- Always have a unique perspective on life to draw from.
- A survivorship care plan may be necessary
- Enjoy support from friends and family
- Frequent checkups with your healthcare providers
- Gradually find a new normal.

Conclusion

Breast diseases, especially breast cancer, have been seen to be a monster that scares the life out of the diagnosed. With an appropriate lifestyle routine that incorporates exercise, diets, and avoidance of smoking and alcohol, a diagnosed patient can live a healthy, happy, and healthy life devoid of morbidity after treatment.